I0409258

Gut Check: The Inside Truth on Restoring Your Digestive Health

# Gut Check: The Inside Truth on Restoring Your Digestive Health

by Robin Terranella, NMD, DiplAcu

Copyright © 2013 Robin Terranella, NMD, DiplAcu. All rights reserved. Printed and bound in the United States of America. No part of this book may be reproduced or transmitted in any form or by any means, electronic or mechanical, including photocopying, recording, or by an information storage and retrieval system – except by a reviewer who may quote brief passages in a review to be printed in a magazine, newspaper, or on the Web – without permission in writing from the author.

Although the author and publisher have made every effort to ensure the accuracy and completeness of information contained in this book, we assume no responsibility for errors, inaccuracies, omissions, or any inconsistency herein. Any slights of people, places, or organizations are unintentional.

Cover Design by Nebojsa Dolovacki
Book Design by Nichole Ward, Morrison Alley Design

First Printing 2013

ISBN 978-1500304409

# TABLE OF CONTENTS

# GUT CHECK: THE INSIDE TRUTH ON RESTORING YOUR DIGESTIVE HEALTH

*Practical information for you to heal your digestive problems naturally.*

You may not know this, but every function of the body is intimately dependent on digestion. Healthy digestion is critical for holistic and optimal health. Your doctors may not have told you how critical your digestive function is to your overall health because they may not connect the dots in the same way a holistic physician does. Or, they may choose not to take the time to deliver this information to you. Whatever the reason, it's critical that you understand how important digestion is for your long term health.

This book will connect those health dots for you and will also show you how to optimize your digestive processes. Whether you suffer from occasional bowel irregularity, gas and/or bloating, or serious and chronic digestive system problems, this book will help you. I am not going to promise you that this will cure every digestive system problem that exists. However, I am confident that you will have better digestion as a result of reading, and implementing, the contents of this book. This Book's premise is to *promote and restore the inherent functions of digestion,* and I have seen these treatments work for hundreds of my own patients.

So, get ready to learn about one of the most important aspects of your health and how to optimize its function.

In this book you will learn:

• The most common problems that can occur with your digestion.

• Background physiology and anatomy to understand why these problems begin in the first place, and how to fix them.

• How to optimize your digestion.

• How to restore vital digestive functions using holistic treatments.

PART 1

# What You Already Know About Digestion

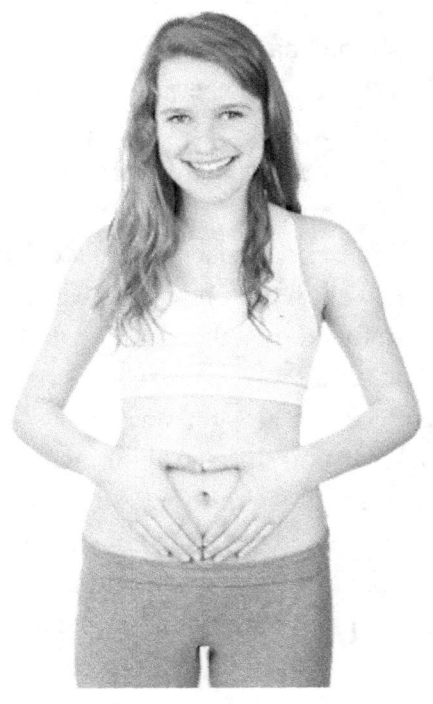

The most straightforward way to understand the problems that arise in your digestive tract is to first look at how "normal digestion" typically works. As I have done throughout www.discoverholistichealth. org, we will start with the things you already know and expand on that knowledge. If you don't think you know anything about your digestion, hang in there; you probably know more than you think. Even though we may not think about *how* it actually works, you have a direct interaction with digestion every day.

## THINGS YOU ALREADY KNOW ABOUT YOUR DIGESTIVE SYSTEM.

Every day you put food in your mouth. This food arrives in various shapes, sizes, and consistencies. Our taste buds are activated as the sweet, salty, sour, spicy, and bland foods enter our mouth. We chew it up - and then swallow it down. At some point in the day (for some of you it may be more like every 2-4 days) you experience how this food changes as it travels through the digestive tract. Can you guess how you experience this change? That's right - in the form of a bowel movement. Some of you may have the unfortunate experience of gas, pains, cramping, diarrhea, and/or bloating, among other symptoms along the way.

These are all direct experiences you have with your digestive system. I am going to show you how you can turn these everyday experiences into useful knowledge about what is going on, and what's *not* going on, inside your digestive system to create these uncomfortable symptoms. **Let's get started!**

Of course, some of you may be thinking, "how is this simple knowledge helpful?" In short, it provides a reference point. It gives you a starting place to build on your knowledge. You know what happens in the beginning, in the end and, in some cases, feelings in the middle. The part(s) that may not be so clear is what happens in between.

Here are some questions that will help you identify what you don't know about digestion yet:

• How does your digestive system transform food?

• What is the purpose of this transformation?

• What problems manifest (as symptoms) in the body when the transformation processes are disrupted?

• What kinds of problems occur in the digestive tract to disrupt the transformation process?

Keep these questions in the forefront of your mind as we unravel more and more information about the digestive process.

## THE PURPOSE OF DIGESTION

In simple terms, **the purpose of digestion** is to extract the micro- and macronutrients out of the food you eat and eliminate the waste. Seems easy enough, right? Conceptually it is easy, but the mechanics of your digestion are actually quite complex. Now that you know the purpose of digestion, would you be able to design a system that fulfills this purpose, extracting nutrients out of the food you eat? What would this system be made of? How would the food get through the system? Try this mental exercise now. Design a system that can extract the nutrition out the food and remove the waste from the system.

You can use analogies from your personal work experience or other areas of your life. Think about your own personal experience with the digestive process and what you already know. Write down your extraction process before moving on.

## LET THE TRANSFORMATION BEGIN

Okay, how did you do? Did you come up with some good ideas to get the nutrition out and remove the waste? Now that you got your brain engaged in this transformation process, let's explore how your body actually performs this process.

The process of digestion can be broken down into two separate actions: the breakdown of food and the absorption of the nutritional components from the food. I like to think of these together as the "extraction process" because the body is literally pulling the nutrition out of the food. It does this in three separate, but related, sections of your body: the stomach, the small intestine, and the large intestine. Each section is responsible for specific parts of the extraction process. You should also know that breakdown and absorption involve many other smaller, yet very crucial, processes. Some of these smaller processes are not covered here.

The extraction process creates the transformation that we are all familiar with. Yet for holistically optimal digestion, each section must perform its responsibilities to its fullest capacity. Let's look at each one separately to see what these responsibilities are.

## FIRST, SOME VERY BASIC ANATOMY

I promise this anatomy lesson will be short and sweet. Your digestive tract is a long narrow tube, made of mostly muscles and separated into different compartments by sphincters. The sphincters only allow the food to travel in one direction. These different compartments each serve different functions in the extraction process. For our purposes, we will talk about three different sections: the stomach, the small intestine, and the large intestine. In sequential order, the mouth feeds into the stomach (orange), the stomach (orange) into the small intestine (orange), the small intestine to the large intestine (green), and the large intestine into the anus (blue).

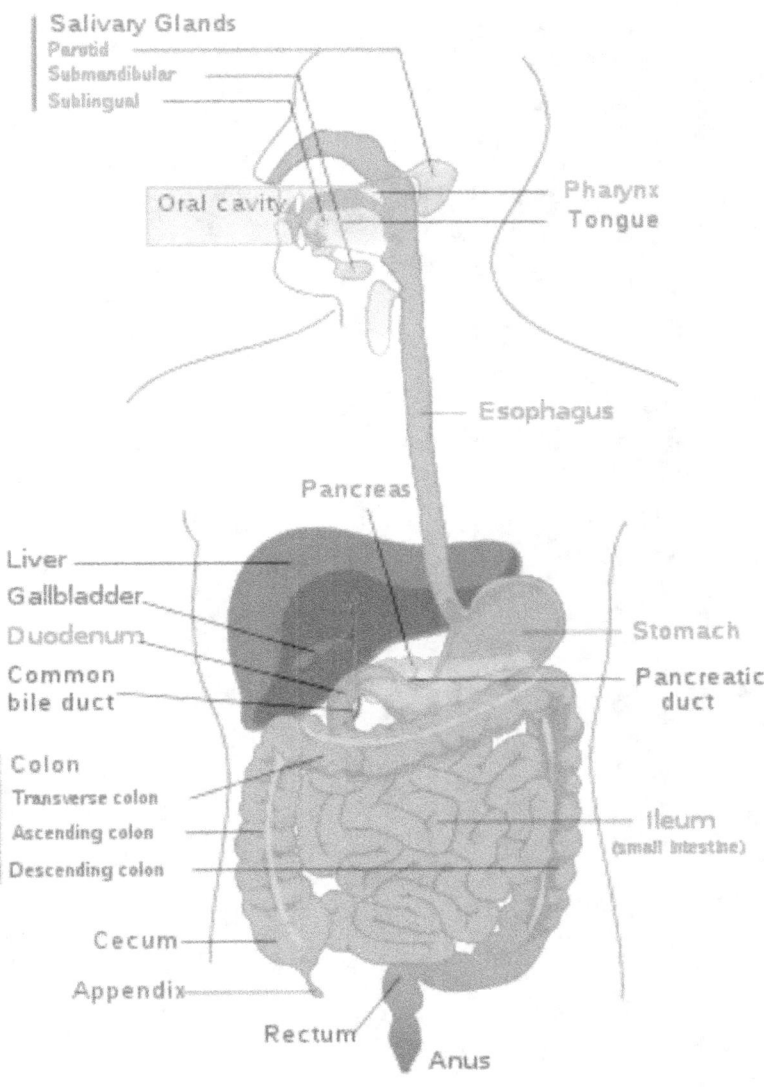

The picture above is a diagram showing each of the different sections that comprise the entire digestive system as a whole. Now let's explore the responsibilities of each in more detail.

# PART 2

# The Individual Actions of Your Digestive Tract

## THE STOMACH.

While digestion actually starts in your mouth, with chewing and saliva, the stomach is where the initial large scale extraction, breakdown and absorption, begins. Most of the action in the stomach is designed to breakdown large food particles into smaller ones. By doing so, it prepares the food for more refined extraction in the small intestine.

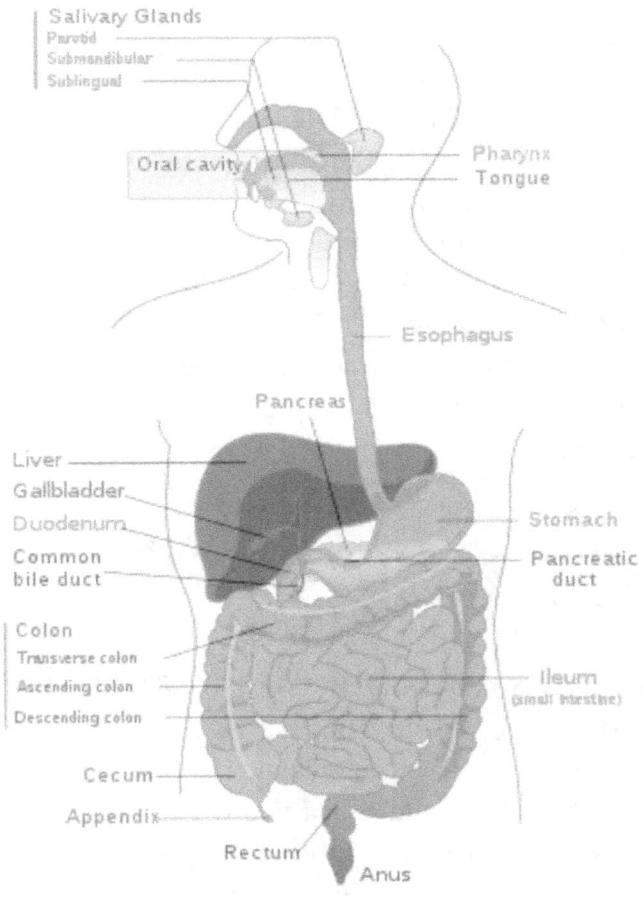

Immediately after you swallow your food, it enters into the stomach and comes into contact with enzymes and acid. The acid is called Hydrochloric acid (HCL) and is produced by cells in the stomach called *parietal cells*. These cells are triggered to secrete HCL when food enters into the stomach and touches them or pushes against them. Even the simple act of smelling mouthwatering food can trigger parietal cells. The acidic HCL substance interacts with the contents of the stomach and does two things:

1.  The HCL breaks down large proteins into smaller ones
2.  The HCL activates enzymes, mainly pepsinogen

The HCL acid itself does a small amount of digestive work on the food in the stomach as well. It performs a function, similar to loosening knots, which is called *denaturing the proteins*. The stomach is a thick muscular sack that churns and mixes the food. Stomach muscles are also activated to start churning when food enters into the stomach and stretches the muscles. In addition to the mechanical action of breaking up the food, the churning action of the stomach brings the HCL into contact with the *pepsinogen*. HCL activates pepsinogen in to *pepsin*. Pepsin is an enzyme that breaks down large proteins into their smaller counterparts, *amino acids* and *peptides.*

**Q: What do you think?**
How long would it take you to breakdown a 6 oz. chicken breast? 10 minutes? 2 hours?

## SIZE MATTERS WHEN IT COMES TO DIGESTION
I am speaking of the size of your...enzymes, in relation to the food, of course. The enzymes that breakdown your food are actually really small. So small, in fact, that in order for them to breakdown solid food, the enzymes have to be constantly mixed with the food to maintain ongoing contact. This mixing process is created by the rhythmic contraction of digestive muscles. This action is called *peristalsis*. In the stomach, this rhythmic movement created by the muscle walls helps activate enzymes, as described above, and also

helps to breakdown the food particles. As the muscles contract, the food particles bang together. This breaks them apart and creates more interaction with the enzymes and acid. The end result is further breakdown of food particles and greater contact with the enzymes.

The combined effort of enzymes and peristalsis changes the shape and structure of the food to prepare it for the next part in the extraction process. The stomach's main purpose is mostly to breakdown the food. The stomach does very little in regards to pulling nutrition out of the food and transferring it into the blood stream, however. That function is highly refined and is a job for the small intestine, which leads perfectly into the next section of the digestive tract.

## THE SMALL INTESTINE HAS A BIG JOB: ABSORPTION, ABSORPTION, ABSORPTION!

Can you guess what the major job of the small intestine is? That's right; absorption *and* extraction. Before that extraction can occur, there is still a large amount of breakdown that must be done simultaneously. Where the stomach left off with protein breakdown, the small intestine picks right up with its own, more refined breakdown process.

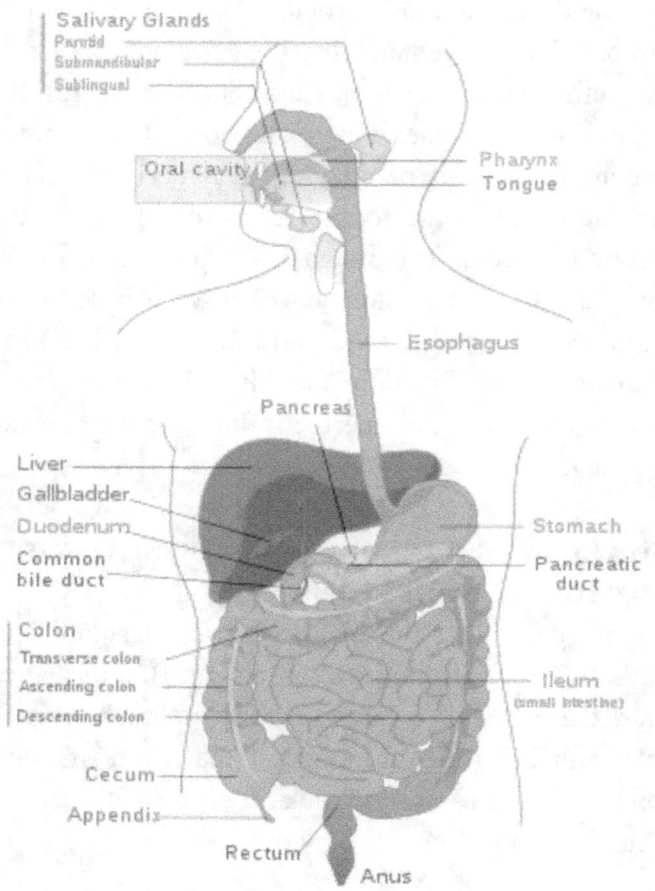

The initial job of the small intestine is to get the incoming food content ready for enzyme action. As the food from the stomach enters into the small intestine, it triggers release of *bicarbonate* from the pancreas. This bicarbonate changes the acidity from high to low – or more alkaline. This change is needed for the newly secreted enzymes to function properly. The enzyme activity in the small intestine is much more diverse than in the stomach. *Lipase* and *protease* are secreted from the pancreas, which breaks down fats and proteins. The presence of fats triggers the gall bladder to contract and secrete bile acids. This bile is critical for absorption and breakdown of fats.

Bile is both water soluble and fat soluble. It separates the fats into smaller sections, allowing the lipase to come into contact with, and breakdown, the fats. Other enzymes, like *maltase*, *amylase*, and *sucrose*, are also part of the digestive tract mucosal layers. These enzymes, and others, are there to help breakdown starches and other plant specific compounds.

Just like the stomach, the small intestine also uses peristalsis, that mixing action, to break the food particles apart and get more enzymes in contact with the food. As this occurs the food particles are broken into smaller and smaller pieces until they are microscopic in size. That's right; the molecules are broken down from bite size to microscopic size. The only thing left to do now is **get the good nutrition into the blood stream and leave the bad stuff behind**.

## LET THE ABSORPTION BEGIN

One of the most incredible things about the small intestine is its ability to pull the nutrients *out* of the food and put them *into* the blood stream. This feat is possible only because of the small intestine's enormous surface area . When viewed simply as a narrow tube with muscles, there is nothing spectacular about it at all. However your small intestine is more than just a narrow tube.

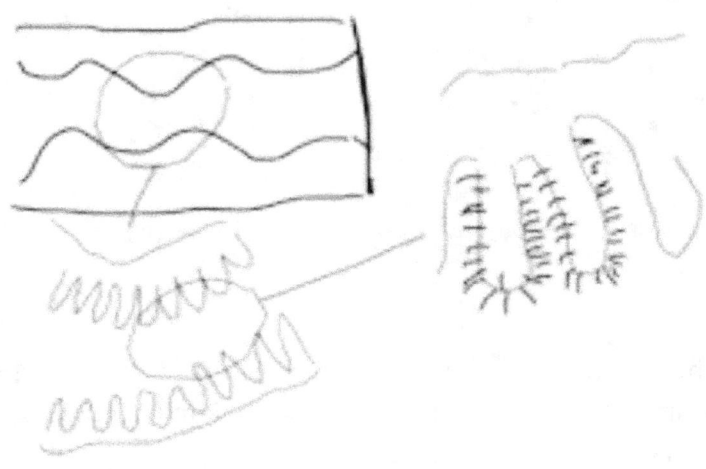

The sketch to the above is intended to illustrate this in its most basic form. The tubular shape of the small intestine is clear but, when you look at it more closely, it also has bump-like projections that jut out into the *lumen* (the insides) of the tube. These bumps are covered by finger-like projections called *villi* and these villi are covered with hair-like projections called *microvilli*. The illustration on the top left is a cross section of a small intestine showing these bump-like projections. Below this are the finger-like projections, the villi. On the right is an illustration of the microvilli, the hair-like projection is located on the villi.

One digestive cell alone may have as many as 10-30 microvilli attached to it. The purpose of the villi and microvilli is to amplify the surface area of the small intestine thousands of times over. This surface area amplification is the key to what makes it possible for nutrients to be pulled out of the food you eat.

Now you may be thinking, **"how do the nutrients get into the body?"**

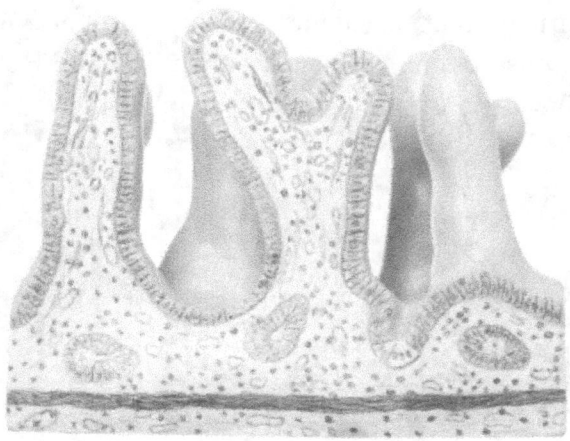

In the illustration above you can see a thin blue line underneath a slightly larger thin pink layer, in addition to sporadic blue spots. This thin pink layer is the microvilli all bunched together. Within the pink layer there are some dark reddish- pink spots. These spots represent the nuclei of individual cells. Below all this you can also see white space, speckled with red dots and lines. These red speckles and lines depict blood vessels. The blood vessels both deliver nutrition to the digestive cells and also take the incoming nutrients away, delivering them to the rest of the body.

When we speak of nutrition, we are referring to both *macronutrients* and *micronutrients*. Macronutrients are comprised of carbohydrates, proteins, and fats. Micronutrients are comprised of vitamins, minerals, plant bioflavonoids, and other nutrients. This nutrition is the basic fuel for each of the cells in our body to stay healthy. Without it we would not be able to function from day to day.

**Q? So how do these nutrients get inside our body's cells? Take a guess.**
**A: Transportation**

As the large food particles turn into smaller and smaller microscopic food particles, they are transported through the microvilli and into the intestinal cells. When the food particles get close enough to the microvilli, they can pass directly through the microvilli and into the corresponding cell. This process is called *diffusion* and there are several different forms of diffusion. The main forms of diffusion are called "active" and "passive" diffusion.

The main process of passive diffusion is quite simple; areas of high particle concentration move to areas of low particle concentration. For some nutrients, energy is used to artificially create the concentration gradient so nutrients can flow into the cell. That is active diffusion. To keep things simple we will stick with the concept of non-energy dependent passive diffusion.

Because each of the smaller microvilli are part of a larger cell, food particles which diffuse into the microvilli must make their way deeper into the cell. Flowing below the cell, opposite the microvilli, are blood vessels. Once the food particles are in the villi, the food particles diffuse through the cell and into the blood stream where they are then transported throughout the body. This is the main way food is transported from the digestive tract into the body.

Another, less utilized, transportation mechanism is for the food particles to pass between the villi, through *gap junctions*, directly into the blood stream. This process accounts for less than 5% of absorption because most of the food particles are too large to fit through these gap junctions. This direct transportation process can be problematic for the body and digestive tract. We will explore these issues in more detail later. Nonetheless, without healthy microvilli, and their corresponding villi, there will be little to no absorption taking place. When food absorption is diminished, due to unhealthy and/or damaged villi and microvilli, there is little to no food or energy available to the rest of the body.

Through this process of breakdown and absorption the nutrients are pulled into the body one-by-one leaving the un-useful food particles behind in the lumen of the small intestine. In time, and as a result of the rhythmic muscle movements, remaining food particles are passed into the large intestine for yet another round of digestion.

## THE LARGE INTESTINE DOES VERY SMALL THINGS.

There is no doubt that the large intestine has many important functions but these functions occur on a smaller level than in the small intestine. When the food from the small intestine is transferred to the large intestine it is in the form of a liquid mush, kind of like the consistency of runny mashed potatoes (yum). At this point in the digestive process, about 90% of the absorption has already occurred.

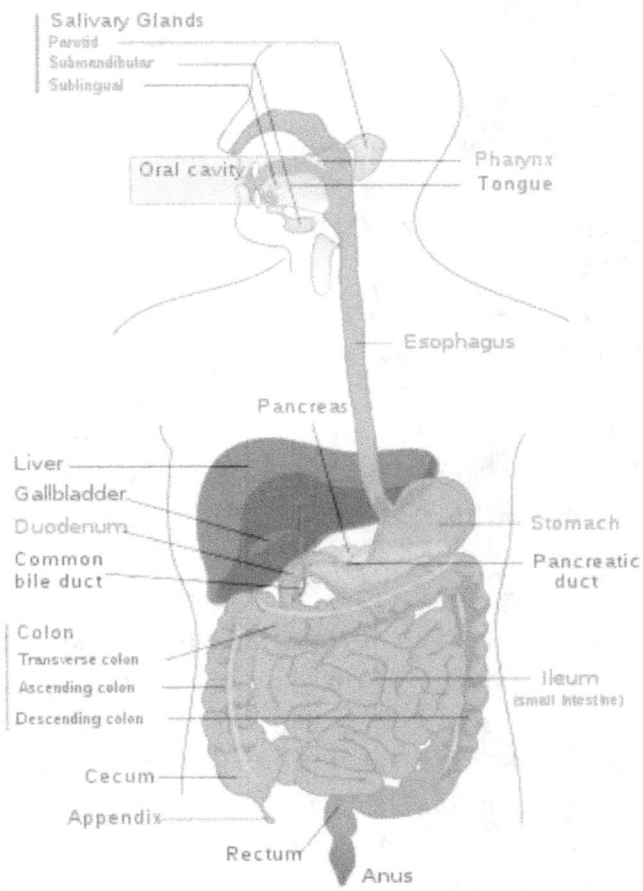

The main responsibilities of the large intestine are:

• fluid reabsorption
• further digestion of complex carbohydrates
• micronutrient production and absorption

Some of these jobs require assistance from the "friendly bacteria" in the large intestine. They are often referred to as *probiotics*. These bacteria play several critical roles in the large intestine, some of which are yet to be fully understood.

## MAKE FRIENDS WITH YOUR NEIGHBORHOOD BACTERIA

Our large intestines are filled with millions of these friendly bacteria. Hundreds of different species and strains come together to create a microscopic ecology, as complex as the rain forest, right in your large intestine. In fact there are more bacteria in you large intestine than cells in your body. The importance of the many different bacterial strains and species is only at the beginning stages of our scientific understanding.

What we do know is that they play critical roles in breaking down complex fibrous food particles, like that found in dark leafy greens, such as Kale. Through this breakdown process, the bacteria make vitamins and micronutrients, like Vitamin K. This is the main source of Vitamin K in our bodies, which is needed for blood clotting factors and bone health. Healthy bacteria also make things like *butyrate,* which is a small chain fatty acid. Butyrate is the desired fuel source for the cells of the large intestine. We will learn more about these friendly bacteria later.

In Part 3 we will explore the following topics with relation to friendly bacteria:
• How specific strains affect the overall balance for food and space.
• The role of these bacteria in immune function.
• How changes in the bacterial ecology can have effects in the skin, sinuses, etc.
• The communication between the intestinal cells and immune system.

## CONTINUING ALONG WITH THE DIGESTIVE PROCESS...

As the remaining food particles travel along through the large intestine, water, sodium, chloride, and magnesium are reabsorbed into the blood stream by *osmosis*. Osmosis is a process similar to passive diffusion. As this liquid material passes further along the large intestine, it becomes more and more solid. Without getting too graphic, you should now have a clear picture of how this transformation takes place. More importantly, **you understand how the process of digestion works -** and soon you'll understand the source of digestive problems and how to fix them.

# PART 3

# How - and Where - Digestion Problems Begin

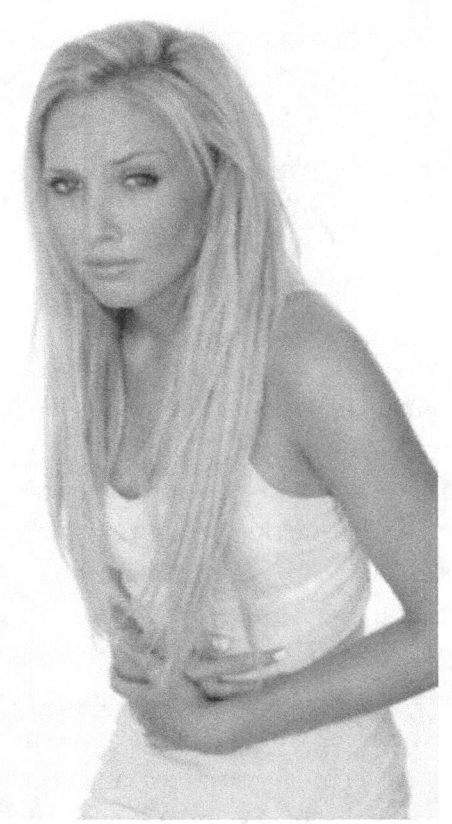

Before we address the problems that can arise during the digestive process, I want you to think back to the process you designed to extract nutrients from your food and eliminate the waste. Now that you have more information at your fingertips, how does your invention compare to the process your body uses? How do your ideas compare to the actual process your body uses. Here is the idea I came up with:

*First off, I thought that to get the nutrition out and leave behind the waste you could use a suctioning device. Kind of like the way you can suck on a popsicle and leave the ice behind. This is sort of what the body is doing in the digestive tract.*

My idea is basic and primitive compared to what is actually happening. Yet, it illustrates the bare bones of what the body does. In order for the body to do this it uses highly refined processes. When these processes are disrupted, problems arise with the extraction process. These problems often show up in predicable patterns, what doctors call "**symptoms and signs**". These patterns of symptoms, and their corresponding treatment(s), will be the focus of the coming sections.

Before we explore these problems, describe how your process was similar and different to the one your body uses. Is it better/worse? Why or why not?

Keep in mind that every single, and seemingly simple, change you could make in the extraction process can have unforeseeable changes in other parts of the body. If we were to change the digestive process by eliminating the enzymes, there would be effects throughout the entire body - not simply in the digestive tract. You can imagine a similar change, such as building a dam in a river. One could easily predict that the river would dry up downstream. But how the dam affects the local ecology 10 miles outside the river bank, both up and down stream, is not easy to predict. In the same way, the body's processes are very much interdependent on one another. With that in mind, *I am going to stick with the digestive process I already have. How about you*?

You may have second thoughts if you suffer with digestive problems, but I have some solutions to help you with these problems. It turns out, if you know what the key areas of digestion are, you have a good chance at fixing them. After all, 75% of treatment hinges on what's causing the problem in the first place. I am going to tell you what the key aspects of digestion are below. It is these players that cause the majority of digestive problems, but first......

See if you can come up with these key areas of digestion on your own. They are covered in the above paragraphs. Use your personal history with eating, and the digestive discomfort you have experienced, to guide you to your answers.

Well, how did you do? Were you able to come up with some of the key players in the extraction process? Let's take a walk through the extraction process from top to bottom and identify them now.

## FOUR KEY AREAS OF DIGESTION

### 1. ENZYMES

Without enzymes there is no breakdown. Without breakdown, there is no absorption, among other things we will explore below.

A lack of digestive enzymes is a common reason for discomfort in your abdomen because your body cannot properly digest food without them. As you might recall, your stomach acid (HCL) is needed to activate these enzymes in your stomach. If you have low acid, the enzymes will not work properly, even if there are plenty of them. When the enzymes do not work, the food you eat, especially the proteins, goes undigested and you feel **bloated, fatigued, and gassy**. So, how do you know if this is an issue for you?

**The telltale signs and symptoms of stomach acid/enzyme deficiency:**

A feeling of fullness after eating only small amounts of food.

• This is because the food you eat is not being digested, or moving through to the stomach. This decreased movement can lead to constipation.

Taking an acid reducing medication.

• This medicine is designed to reduce the amount of irritation and inflammation caused by stomach acid, but the reduced acid comes with a price: poor digestion. If you can get away with not taking them, you will be better off in the future. *However, you should consult a healthcare provider before doing so.*

Feeling like the food just seems to sit there.

• This occurs because the food *is* just sitting there and not moving to the second phase of digestion in the small intestine.

Fatigue after meals

• This happens because the body is using so much energy to digest the food there is little left for your daily activities. Plus, you are not getting all the micro and macro nutrients out of the food.

Gas in the form of belching or otherwise

• Gas occurs for two reasons; the first reason is from swallowed air during eating. This is normal and usually forms a burp. The second reason is from poorly digested food. This occurs because as bacteria in the digestive system interact with undigested carbohydrates, they ferment the food, creating gas. When food is improperly digested by the acid and enzymes, more gas is created. **Acid blocker anyone?**

Since the digestive process is like an assembly line, the incomplete breakdown of food in the stomach is transferred to the small intestine. As with any factory, when the previous worker did not do their job, the next in line cannot do their job either. The food that enters the small intestine will not be as liquefied and will remain a minimally digested mass of food. In order for the small intestine to provide the same level of absorption it normally would, the enzymes have to work extra hard. The muscles involved in peristalsis would also have to work extra hard. I don't think I have to tell you that **the small intestine is not designed to do the work of the stomach.** The end result is poor absorption and the resulting low energy from poor nutrition.

In some cases of low stomach acid, the muscles that line the stomach will try to compensate by using increased *peristalsis,* that churning action, for longer periods of time. This can lead to nausea, cramps, and stomach pain, as well as constipation.

Can you guess what would happen from low or inadequate enzyme amounts in the small intestine? You guessed it: **Poor absorption.**

## SO YOU THINK YOU HAVE LOW STOMACH ACID/ ENZYME SECRETION... NOW WHAT?

If you think you suffer from low stomach acid or enzyme production, you are in luck. I am going to share several ways for you to improve these functions. Each option will allow for greater enzyme / acid secretion. Your goal should be *adequate* enzyme/acid secretion as too much secretion can also cause irritation and damage to the mucosa of the stomach and esophagus. The idea is to provide just enough for full breakdown of food.

### Option One:

Take a lemon, slice it, and squeeze the juice into about 4-6 ounces of water. Alternatively, you can use vinegar or lemon juice concentrate. Before each major meal (lunch and dinner - or all three if you eat a good sized breakfast), you will want to drink this solution. Start with 1/2 a lemon (or 1 teaspoon of vinegar) and see if it helps your symptoms over the course of 3-5 days. If this doesn't seem to be alleviating the symptoms above, work your way up to a full lemon or even 2 lemons in water before major meals. If it still does not work, move on to option 2. If it seems to make things worse, you may need to work on repairing the mucosa first (see below,under the heading "Mucosa").

### How it works

The acid in lemons (or vinegar) is similar to HCL and will help activate digestive enzymes. When the food enters your mouth and then the stomach, those enzymes will be raring to go and able to digest the proteins efficiently.

---

### TIP: Don't drink a lot of liquid with meals

*Drinking more than a cup of water or tea with meals dilutes stomach acid making you less able to digest your foods. Instead drink 15-20 minutes before starting your meal.*

---

## Option Two:

Need more help with digestive function? If the first option didn't seem to do the trick, or if you think you could use more help, you will need to go out and purchase some HCL tablets (*note: they should be in tablet form **not** capsule*).

Many of the products on the market have additives in addition to HCL. Try to find a product with pure HCL. It may come in the form of betaine HCL, which is equally as beneficial as HCL. Take about 500-1500mg with your larger meals. It is best to take this right before, or right after, you have begun your meal.

Please note that this can cause nausea and intense burning in the stomach if you take too much, or on an empty stomach. It is advised to start with 500mg first and work up to larger doses as tolerated or as needed. If your symptoms are not alleviated or improved by the HCL tablets within five days, consider moving to option three.

## Option Three:

If you think you still need further help in this capacity, your third option is to purchase a digestive enzyme and HCL blend. Remember, proteases are the main enzymes in the stomach. Lipase, amylase, trypsinogen, and others come from the pancreas and are important to the small intestine. These additional enzymes can help when your body is not making enough of its own necessary enzymes. As with the above, you should start with a low dose first and work your way up.

If you suffer from low energy, indigestion during or after meals, or gas and bloating during or after meals, then poor digestion may be the culprit. If it is, you will notice an improvement in most of these symptoms after starting on any of the above regimens. If low energy is a major health issue for you, you can expect an increase in energy within about 2-3 weeks' time. As the increased digestion allows for increased nutritional extraction, these nutrients will be delivered throughout the cells of the body. Most people will gradually notice this increase in energy over the coarse of 2 weeks.

## 2. MUCOSA

**Greater surface area means greater absorption. How great is that?**

The mucosa of your digestive tract is a thin layer of cells that interact with the food particles in the lumen of the stomach and intestines. The diagram above, showing the villi and microvilli in the small intestine, is an example of the mucosa in the small intestine. This thin layer of cells secretes mucus that serves as a protective barrier against the enzymes and acids that are secreted for digestion. This layer is also responsible for transferring the nutrients from the lumen of the digestive tract into the blood. Dysfunction and/or damage in this layer of cells leads to poor absorption of nutrients. This makes sense since the food particles have to pass through these cells to enter into the blood. **So what types of dysfunction can arise and how does this come about?**

When we refer to "dysfunction" we are referring to a collective damage and/or inadequate function in the mucosal layer and/or group of cells. This dysfunction comes about for various reasons:
• Inflammation
• Poor Nutrient Absorption/Consumption
• Chronic Inflammatory Insults

Even small amounts of damage to the villi and microvilli can really impair the absorption process. As previously mentioned, most of the absorption of your nutrients occurs in the small intestine. It is therefore more damaging to the entire body when the mucosal dysfunction occurs in the small intestine, versus the stomach or large intestine. Still, damaging dysfunction in the mucosal layer can occur in any part of the digestive tract. That said, we will focus on the ways the dysfunction presents itself in the small intestine, since this is the most crucial area for absorption.

## INFLAMMATION

Your immune system uses inflammation as a tool to protect it from foreign invaders and to repair damage that occurs anywhere in the body. In the mucosa of the small intestine, inflammation occurs when immune cells detect a food allergen or pathogenic bacteria. Food allergens and sensitivities are the most common trigger of inflammation in the small intestine.

Your immune system is like a security system that responds to threats by sending messages to its counterparts (other immune cells). These messages tell the immune cells to attack and isolate any foreign invader - both locally, in the digestive tract, and systemically. The strategy of the immune system is to isolate the threat and prevent it from spreading further in the body. This is similar to what would occur with any security system. However, these attacks and isolation methods can eventually lead to tissue damage in the digestive tract, or wherever it occurs.

Occasional, or infrequent, inflammation and ensuing tissue damage presents very few problems. However, with daily occurrence, the mucosa has no way to regenerate and rebuild. In this case the mucosa is constantly inflamed and lacks critical microvilli.

The amount of mucosal damage can vary greatly:
• Damage to the microvilli
• Mild inflammation in the microvilli or villi
• Full blown ulcers that erode the entire villi, neighboring villi, and more.

In all of the cases above, the end result is a decrease in the absorptive capabilities of the small intestine. As you might predict, the greater the tissue damage the more damage to the absorptive capabilities. To illustrate this, think back to the analogy we made about the absorption function of the small intestine. If the function of the small intestine is similar to a vacuum that pulls out the desired nutrients and leaves behind the waste, what happens when there are less microvilli and villi?

You see, the microvilli and villi are like the power behind this vacuum. When we take away only some of the microvilli, it significantly reduces the absorptive power. It would be like using an old model vacuum that is powered by pushing the vacuum across the floor rather than by electricity. This is why even small amounts of damage lead to large changes in absorption. In many of these cases of mucosal damage and or inflammation, *the foods you eat are the cause of the damage. Below we will discuss the solution to this potential problem.*

## POOR NUTRIENT ABSORPTION / CONSUMPTION

Not only does what you eat contribute to inflammation, poor eating habits can limit the ability of the villi and microvilli to regrow and repair damaged areas. The microvilli of the mucosa are constantly being recycled and regenerated into new fresh mucosa. In fact, this is one of the most rapidly regenerating areas of your body. The mucosa regenerates every couple of days but it requires adequate vitamins to do so. The required vitamins are folic acid, b12, and b6. The interesting thing about the relationship between these vitamins and microvilli growth is that without microvilli, absorption of b12, folic acid, and b6 is very difficult. Yet without the vitamins the microvilli cannot regenerate. It is a conundrum. While it's not an impossible situation, this conundrum makes mucosal repair difficult to overcome (see below, *"What can I do to help protect, minimize, and/or reverse inflammation in my mucosa?"*, for more details on how to overcome this damage).

Chronic alcohol consumption is a real life example of how mucosal damage can manifest from vitamin deficiency. Alcohol consumption causes our bodies to excrete vitamins through our urine ( in particular B vitamins). Over time, vitamin deficiencies will lead to decreased villi and microvilli growth. The lack of microvilli leads to poor absorption and further vitamin deficiencies. A similar cyclical situation occurs with poor nutrition and vitamin intake.

## CHRONIC INFLAMMATORY INSULTS

With repeated insults, chronic inflammation in the mucosa will cause ulcerations in the mucosa itself. The reason(s) this occurs are different based on the area of the digestive tract in which it occurs. In the small intestine, food allergies, pathogenic bacteria, food sensitivities, *dysbiosis* (microbial imbalances in the body), genetic predispositions, and autoimmune conditions play the biggest roles.

## FOOD ALLERGIES AND SENSITIVITIES

Food allergies and food sensitivities, create inflammatory patterns based on the reaction of the immune system. The pattern starts with the immune system's recognition of a foreign invader passing through the mucosal cells. This recognition triggers the immune cells to send signals to other immune cells locally and systemically. These signals tell the immune cells what the foreign invader looks like and where to find it. In the case of a food allergy, these signals lead to a quick and dramatic isolation of the invader. It also creates a host of severe allergic symptoms ranging from abdominal pain and wheezing, to hives and anaphylactic shock. The good thing is that the immune cells protect the body from these foreign invaders. Unfortunately, with food allergies, the immune response to the allergens can be so severe that major tissue damage occurs. In some cases, food allergies can result in death, like in the case of a severe peanut allergy, which demonstrates the effectiveness of the immune response.

On the other hand, food sensitivities cause local and systemic immune responses that have less dramatic, and less immediate, consequences. These smaller responses by the immune system often go unnoticed because of the delayed and subdued symptoms they create. Yet, when repeated on a daily basis, they too can lead to chronic inflammation and damage to the mucosa, as mentioned above.

## PATHOGENIC BACTERIA AND DYSBIOSIS

Pathogenic bacteria and dysbiosis can also create a similar pattern of inflammation and mucosal damage. The hundreds of strains of bacteria in the colon exist in a delicate balance. Even the pathogenic and bad bacteria are a normal part of your colonic flora. In some cases the flora can become out of balance, allowing the pathogenic bacteria to replicate and overpopulate. This overpopulation triggers the immune system to respond and reestablish balance. So, inflammation *and* pathogenic bacteria damage the mucosa.

A classic example of this process occurs with the bacteria *Clostridium difficile* (aka *C. diff.*). These pathogenic bacteria can overpopulate the colon when people are given antibiotics. Antibiotics are not discretionary: they kill the good bacteria along with the bad bacteria in your body. As antibiotics kill many of the healthy strains of bacteria in the colon, it leaves certain strains of bacteria in greater numbers than the local ecology is used to. The most common antibiotics that cause *C. diff* are ampicillin, amoxicillin, and cephalosporin. Other antibiotics can cause *C. diff* as well, but these antibiotics are more likely to kill the friendly bacteria and not the *C. diff*. The topic of the flora and bacteria in the colon is discussed further below. As the good bacteria are killed off, *Clostridium difficile* overpopulate the flora of the colon. These bacteria can destroy the mucosa and the immune system is triggered to fight them off.

## AUTOIMMUNE AND GENETICS

Another cause for mucosal damage is from a group of conditions collectively referred to as IBD (Irritable Bowel Disease). The exact mechanism of how and why they occur is not completely understood, but we do know that family history and genetics play a role. With IBD the mucosa is damaged by the immune system in a fashion that is thought to be autoimmune in nature. The basic mechanism of how the damage occurs is similar to the process of the immune cells responding to an allergen. In the case of autoimmune disease, the immune cells falsely see the digestive cells as a foreign invader. This causes the immune cells to attack and destroy these "foreign" cells. The patterns of damage will vary, depending on which IBD (Crohn's, Ulcerative Colitis, Celiac's Disease, etc.) you have. Even though these are not classically thought of as being caused by food sensitivities, it has been my experience that certain foods do affect them. More information about this will be provided in the treatment section below.

## SO HOW DO YOU KNOW IF YOU HAVE A PROBLEM WITH YOUR DIGESTIVE MUCOSA?

One way to tell if your digestive system is suffering from a mucosal issue is by paying attention to the signs and symptoms of your body. Signs are physical attributes, like diarrhea, and symptoms are subjective things, like abdominal pain. Both signs and symptoms are like clues that help you identify what is going on inside your body since you cannot see inside there. Let's look at some of these clues in more depth.

Pain can be a vague symptom, but it does tell us that there is some degree of inflammation present. Mucosal damage is not the only cause of abdominal pain, however, it is one of the most common causes of it.. When the pain is severe, the inflammation is likely to be more severe too. The frequency of pain can also be an indication of severity. For instance, if the pain is a daily occurrence, there is more of an issue than if it is an occasional discomfort. If the pain is accompanied by blood or mucus in your stool, this is a more extreme clue and typically reflects even more damage to the mucosa.

*Note: Bright red blood in the toilet often results from hemorrhoids and constipation rather than IBD. However, in either case, you should consult with a health professional.*

An additional sign of mucosal damage is loose stools and / or diarrhea. When these result from mucosal damage it is usually after severe and ongoing mucosal damage. As the food passes through the small intestine and cannot be absorbed, it is pushed into the colon.

Other, more general, symptoms that result from poor absorption of nutrients are fatigue, poor sleep, headaches, weak brittle hair and fingernails, etc. These signs are reflective of poor digestion and absorption, but can result from other things besides mucosal damage.

A biopsy of the intestines in a person with Irritable Bowel Disease clearly shows mucosal damage. The symptoms that accompany these conditions are usually abdominal pain, diarrhea, mucus in stool, and blood in the stool. Blood in the stool will usually appear dark or black in color but could also be bright red. Luckily there are holistic treatments that can help resolve this damage without using harsh medications.

In some cases medications are needed to resolve digestive issues. However there are simple things that can be done to make a remarkable difference *without* the use of medication. If you are already on medications, you should know that these treatments can be used in conjunction with conventional medical treatments.

## WHAT CAN I DO TO HELP PROTECT, MINIMIZE, AND/ OR REVERSE INFLAMMATION IN MY MUCOSA?

There are three main things you can do to minimize and reverse inflammation and damage to the mucosa;
• Maintain proper balance of fatty acids
• Remove triggers
• Ingest sufficient and proper vitamins and minerals

The most effective, and probably the most challenging, of these is to remove the triggers. As you will see, using a specific plan and some persistence, you can easily accomplish all of the above.

## BALANCE OF FATTY ACIDS

The food you eat plays a big role in the amount of inflammation your body creates. In fact, you can reduce the amount of inflammation your body produces by reducing the inflammatory fuel it has access to. That's right; your body needs fuel for inflammation and that fuel is omega 6 fatty acids.

When the amount of omega 6 fatty acids greatly outweighs the amount of omega 3 fatty acids, your body is more prone to creating inflammation when damage occurs. Most Americans eat more omega 6 than omega 3 by a ratio of 8:1 and some experts approximate it at numbers even higher than that. When the cells in the digestive tract are damaged, they produce molecules that can either be *anti*-inflammatory or *pro*-inflammatory. When the cells are made of mostly omega 3 fatty acids they produce anti-inflammatory molecules. When your cells are made of mostly omega 6 fatty acids they produce pro- inflammatory molecules. The optimal dietary balance of omega 6 to omega 3 is about a 3:1 ratio. Your body still needs more omega 6 than omega 3 but certainly not eight to twelve times more.

This means about 1/3 of your unsaturated fat calories should be from omega 3 fatty acids: fish, nuts, seeds, grass fed beef, other sea foods. The other 2/3 from non-omega 3 sources such as omega 6 and 9 fatty acids. To put this in perspective, the average American diet has almost zero omega 3 fatty acids. So changing 1/3 of your unsaturated fat calories to omega 3 is a big increase for most people. For comparison's sake, a 1200 calorie diet would equate to consuming about 6 grams of total omega 3 for the day. Most of us get about 30% of calories from fat. For 1200 calories, that would be 360 calories. About 1/2 to 2/3 of that will be from saturated fats, leaving about 180 calories for unsaturated fats. If 1/3 of this is from omega 3 sources, that gives us 6 grams/day. That is a significant dose of omega 3 but not all that significant when compared to the overall fats consumed.

It should be noted that your omega 3 sources should have EPA and DHA. You can think of EPA and DHA like the active omega 3 fatty acids since this is where most of the know and desired biological activity comes from. The amount of EPA should be greater than the DHA for decreasing inflammation. If you are consuming 6 grams of omega 3, about 1/2 to 2/3 should be EPA.

## REMOVE TRIGGERS

The other source of inflammation and mucosal damage comes from consuming foods that cause - or trigger - mucosal damage, and therefore an immune response. Food allergens, or food sensitivities, are high on that list. These food triggers are more common than you might think. As foods pass through the mucosa, your immune system is triggered when it detects large foreign proteins (peptides) trying to enter into the blood stream. Once a peptide is detected by an immune cell, the cell will make antibodies *against* the peptide and send signals to other immune cells to help isolate the peptide. This isolation and destruction process leads to damage and inflammation of the mucosal cells, as well as the peptide. The mucosa can recover from this when the damage is occasional. However, when you continuously consume foods that trigger an immune response, and foreign proteins are constantly being detected, the inflammation and antibodies it creates become chronic. The chronic inflammation makes recovery more difficult, and destruction of villi more prominent. Not only does this chronic process destroy digestive function but it also becomes more likely that antibodies will cross-react with self-proteins. This process is called *autoimmunity* (see below for more details on correlation with autoimmunity).

In a repetitive fashion, the original cell(s) that detected the foreign peptide(s) will replicate, passing on the memory of this foreign peptide to its offspring. Next time the same peptide tries to enter the blood stream, the new immune cells will release antibodies, and chemical messengers, to isolate and destroy the peptide(s). The next time the response will be even greater, more rapid, and farther reaching in the body. The resulting inflammation causes destruction of the microvilli and even ulceration in some cases. In this way the body can become more and more sensitive to certain foods as it comes in contact with them more often.

It is not the contact foods have within the digestive tract that causes this sensitivity. The sensitivities occur when large food particles, particularly proteins, are absorbed through the gaps in digestive cells into the body. These proteins are what trigger an immune response. If the immune response triggers antibody production, the antibodies can cross-react with the proteins in your body. The cross reaction occurs when the incoming proteins have a similar structure as certain tissues in your body, like joints, thyroid, and other tissues.

If this occurs, each time you eat that particular food you will have a local immune attack against the food and a systemic reaction in the tissues where the antibodies have cross reactivity. Inflammation and immune response tends to perpetuate the problem, leading to *leaky gut syndrome*.

Leaky gut syndrome refers to the process whereby large peptides and proteins pass into the blood stream before they are properly broken down. Leaky gut syndrome commonly occurs in individuals with inflamed digestive tracts. When digestive inflammation occurs, the gaps between the digestive cells, known as gap-junctions, expand. The expansion allow larger peptides and proteins to enter directly into the blood stream rather than via diffusion. As more peptides and proteins seep in, more inflammation occurs. So, food allergies, food sensitivities, and inflammation can actually create more problems if not controlled.

The trick is to figure out which foods your immune system is reacting to and remove them from your diet. To do this you will need to do an elimination diet, which we will explore in more detail below. *Note: food sensitivities can be tested for in the blood but it* *can be expensive ($200 or more) and is not as accurate  following the elimination diet precisely.*

## THE ELIMINATION DIET PROCESS

The elimination diet is the diet used to identify which foods your digestive system and immune system may be reacting to. While we typically use this diet to address digestive problems in the small intestines and colon, it can be sued for any digestive problem you might have. The basic process is quite simple. First, completely eliminate all potential food sensitivities from your diet (see below for a detailed list of most common food sensitivities). It is important that food sensitivities are eliminated 100% for the entire three to eight weeks.  This gives the immune system a chance to down regulate and become less reactive to the foods. You follow this diet for a minimum of three weeks and maximum of eight weeks. During this time, you will often see a regression of many digestive, and other, symptoms you might have. If you don't see an improvement in symptoms, continue with the diet and work on mucosal repair.

After three to eight weeks on the diet, you will be ready to test the foods you have been avoiding one at a time. If you make it 3 weeks and you still have symptoms, continue until your symptoms start to go away for a maximum of 8 weeks. To do this with the most accuracy, it is advised that you:

1.  Read labels carefully to make sure you are only consuming items on the list of allowable foods. To this end, it is best that you prepare all your own foods. although it is possible to eat prepared foods if you are savvy about ingredients.

 a.  See book "An A-Z Guide to Food Additives: Never Eat What You Can't Pronounce."

2.  Keep a small notebook and keep track of everything you eat, during the entire challenge process.

3. Note the time and date, when you actually challenge a food.

4. Note any symptoms that come about over the 48 hrs after each challenge. The symptoms don't have to be isolated to the digestive tract.

5. If symptoms of any kind emerge during the challenge process, that is a positive finding. You will need to avoid this food for the remainder of the challenge process.

6. If no symptoms emerge after 48 hours, you can re-incorporate the food into your diet as you continue to challenge foods.
Continue testing foods after 48 hrs.

It is very important to keep good and accurate records and be diligent when testing foods. Many people will follow the diet perfectly and when it comes time to challenge, they say "I just want to eat in this restricted way from now on." While it is a good diet, this is not realistic and highly discouraged until after challenging. Most people will not be able to maintain this diet and eventually "cheat". Eventually you end up right back where you were, with no idea what caused your symptoms. So, diligence and accuracy are important in the successful completion of the elimination diet.

Once you have tested all foods go back through your records and see what you can and cannot eat. Any foods which caused noticeable symptoms should be avoided for at least six months. If the symptoms were mild, you can test this food again after a six month hiatus. If the symptoms were moderate, you can test it again in nine months. If the symptoms were severe you can test it again in about 12-18 months. Once you re-test a food, you may be able to eat it on a semi-regular basis, once weekly, or once monthly, depending on whether or not symptoms re-emerge. The foods that caused a strong reaction should be avoided completely. It is possible that by avoiding the trigger food(s) for long enough, and following the mucosal repair recommendations below, you will be able to eat your trigger food(s) again.

## ELIMINATION DIET FOOD LIST

### Foods to avoid
- Gluten (Wheat, Barley, Rye, Spelt)
- Dairy
- Eggs
- Corn (including high fructose corn syrup)
- Sugar
- Citrus
- Nightshades (tomatoes, eggplant, peppers, potatoes)
- Soy
- Peanuts
- Beef, Chicken, Turkey, Pork

### Foods to continue
- Beans
- Lamb
- All vegetables (except Nightshades and corn)
- All fruit (except citrus)
- Maple syrup and stevia

## PROPER VITAMINS AND MINERALS: MUCOSAL REPAIR

The last aspect of repairing mucosal damage is related to delivering enough specific vitamins and minerals needed by the mucosa. As we mentioned above B12, B6, and folic acid are required for the villi and microvilli to regenerate. If you have damage to your mucosa, you will need more than an average person to regenerate these areas. There are oral supplements you can take for all three of these vitamins. Sublingual, or under the tongue, forms are best for ideal absorption. By placing the vitamins under the tongue they can be absorbed directly by the capillary system that is located underneath the tongue. The oral vitamin dose should be as follows:
- 1000 mcg B12, 1-2 times daily for 2-4 weeks.
- 100 mg B 6 1 time, daily for 2-4 weeks.
- 400-800 mcg Folic Acid, 1-2 times daily for 2-4 weeks.

Other nutrients important for digestive system health:

• **L Glutamine** - This amino acid helps to catalyze the repair of any damaged small intestine mucosal cells and lining. 2-3 grams twice daily is a good starting dose. This can be increased to 5-7 grams/day.

• **Fish Oil (Omega 3s)** - As mentioned above, this can decrease the amount of pro- inflammatory molecules produced when damage occurs. By lowering the inflammatory response, further damage will be minimized and current damage will be quelled. The suggested dose is 3-4 grams of total omega 3. This can also be increased slowly to 6-8 grams. Your omega 3 content should contain EPA which is the most important omega 3 fatty acid for decreasing inflammation. Of the 4 grams/day at least 1.5 grams should be EPA.

• **Coconut Oil** - Made of mostly medium chain triglycerides, this oil actually feeds the *enterocytes,* digestive system cells. It also soothes and coats the lining, calming any inflammation and damage that might be present. This is particularly important for the colonic mucosa, since the cells and bacteria here regularly feed on medium chain triglycerides in the form of butyrate.

• **Slippery Elm (Ulmus officionalis)** - This herb can be used as a tea or you can get capsules of extract. It works by soothing the mucus membranes throughout the digestive lining and increasing the protective mucus that covers the digestive cells.

• **Probiotics** - These are discussed in detail below (under colonic bacteria)

## 3. PERISTALSIS / NERVOUS SYSTEM

Remember that peristalsis is the act of muscular contraction in the digestive tract that rhythmically pushes the food along, and aides in the digestive process. Because it is a key aspect of digestion, problems with peristalsis create problems with digestion.

This process of peristalsis is controlled by both your local and central nervous systems. If the stimulation for peristalsis is not functioning properly, it can derail the entire digestive process, leading to problems like Irritable Bowel Syndrome (IBS). Let's explore the process and controls of peristalsis to give us a better understanding of how a derailing might occur.

Peristalsis is controlled mainly by the local nervous system in the digestive tract, called the enteric nervous system, and partially by the central nervous system. The muscles running throughout the digestive tract are numerous and are arranged in two separate directions: lengthwise and circularly. The main stimulus for these muscles to contract is the stretching that occurs when food enters into the digestive tract. The stretch receptors are connected to the enteric nervous system, which is activated by the entrance of food. The more stretch, the more activation and resulting peristalsis. So the enteric nervous system is mostly self-contained in this fashion. However, there *is* input to the enteric nervous system from the central nervous system.

The role of the central nervous system comes in the form of the *autonomic nervous system*. The autonomic nervous system can act as a primer for peristalsis activity. Meaning, it can enhance or inhibit both the peristalsis activity and the enzyme secretions created by the enteric nervous system.

The autonomic nervous system is a smaller subset of the central nervous system and it has two parts, *parasympathetic* and *sympathetic*. The parasympathetic is the part that allows for, and enhances, digestion. The sympathetic inhibits digestion. In medical school we remembered it like this; "parasympathetic is "rest and digest", and sympathetic is "fight or flight."

As you can imagine, too much sympathetic stimulation will cause the process of digestion to slow or shut down. When the sympathetic system is stimulated it shifts the body's energy away from digestion and towards physical activity, movement, and stimulation. This means blood flow and energy is diverted away from digestion and toward the heart and muscles of the body. When this occurs, the digestive system can only rely on the enzymes and peristalsis created by the enteric nervous system by the presence of food.

The end result of excess sympathetic activity during digestion is poor breakdown and absorption of your food. Increased sympathetic activity also causes an increase in peristalsis in the large intestine. Most people notice this as an urgency to have a bowl movement when they are nervous or under a lot of stress. On the other hand, parasympathetic activity not only increases peristalsis and blood flow to the digestive tract, it also stimulates digestive enzyme secretion.

In general, we can say that most of the issues arising from peristalsis have to do with a dysfunction in the autonomic nervous system. The issues mainly arise when people with this dysfunction eat food while they are under stress. The presence of food in the digestive tract will causes peristalsis from the stretching action, but the sympathetic drive from stress causes peristalsis to shut down. So it is almost like tug of war from both sides of the nervous system. This leads to cramping and pain from the incomplete and constant contractions. When this occurs, the food will not move at all, and the person will be constipated with cramps and bloating.

Some researchers have characterized this issue as *visceral hypersensitivity*. It has been hypothesized that this visceral hypersensitivity is triggered by food sensitivities and allergies. Others maintain it is simply an excess in sympathetic drive in the nervous system causing disruption in digestion In either case the result is undigested food in the stool and an urgency to evacuate the bowels during, or immediately after, meals. This alternation of constipation and diarrhea is a characteristic of IBS.

## HOW DO I KNOW IF I HAVE AN ISSUE WITH PERISTALSIS?

The symptoms described above can give you some clues into the issues that can arise from problems with peristalsis. The main digestive condition that occurs with dysfunctional peristalsis is IBS.

People with IBS can suffer from any of the following:
• Cramping and/or pain
• Regular or frequent diarrhea or loose stools
• Constipation (having less than one bowel movement daily)
• Gas and bloating
• Fatigue
• Abdominal pain that is relieved by bowel movements

IBS is usually classified as either IBS-d (for diarrhea) or IBS-c (for constipation). While most people with IBS tend toward having either constipation or diarrhea, both are usually present to some degree.  However, the majority of people have IBS-d. In either case, IBS is thought to stem, in part, from the enteric and autonomic nervous system and its relation to the peristaltic activity.

While the above symptoms pertain to IBS, they can also be accompanying symptoms of other digestive conditions. It is also possible to experience these symptoms without having IBS or any significant digestive problem. For instance, your symptoms could be from the occasional digestive irregularity that occurs with diet changes, activity levels, or lifestyle changes. To know for sure, you should consult with a health care professional.

## WHAT CAN I DO TO MINIMIZE PROBLEMS WITH PERISTALSIS?

The problems that arise with peristalsis can be improved by improving the functions of the central and autonomic nervous system. Peristalsis is a function mostly controlled through the nervous system. As such, one primary consideration should be your general mental state, how you respond to and manage stress, and - in particular - your mental state before and around eating. Are you eating on the go? Are you thoroughly chewing your foods?

———————

*"Chew your drink and drink your food"* - Thich Nhat Hanh

———————

Mental state plays a big role in the activity of your central nervous system. This can be more difficult to grasp then you may think. As you sit there reading this, you may say, "I am not stressed", or "I don't feel stress when I am eating."

I would say, "pay closer attention". We all experience stress in our lives. Stress comes when the world we see, feel, and hear is different than our expectations. When the world does not unfold to our expectations, we experience stress. Most of us spend our days trying to adjust, or change, the world around us to make it fit with how we want or expect it to be. When these attempts are working in our favor, there is less stress, but when these attempts are not going in our favor it can become stressful to the point of acute anxiety and depression.

How do you think your nervous system responds during all of this mental and physical activity? Most of the time, the nervous system stays active even after the physical activity is over. This is because those events are being played over and over again in the mind. In order for your body to relax and digest you have to remove those reverberations from your body and mind. This activity in your nervous system is often subconscious, so you may not feel or notice it outright. The more you pay attention, the more it will become obvious to you.

If you are eating while working, driving, or during any other activity, you will have a higher level of sympathetic activity in your body than if you are just sitting and eating. This corresponding activity will alter the stimulation to the digestive system muscles. If you are sitting, eating, and worrying about the project you have to do, these mental activities *also* alter the stimulation to the digestive muscles. Even though you *think* you may not be stressed, sometimes you really have to focus on relaxation in order to get into a parasympathetic state.

As we reviewed above, the process of digestion requires parasympathetic stimulation - which coincides with relaxation and rest. With this in mind, I always recommend that my patients, especially those with digestive issues, take five minutes before eating to relax, in order to optimize their digestion. You can use any method that works for you. The important part is that you actually do it. The bonus for doing this, besides what I've mentioned, is that some of these relaxation techniques will carry over into your other daily activities, which should promote more peace in your life. If you don't have a relaxation method, here are some examples of my favorite techniques:

**1. Deep abdominal awareness breathing** – take a deep breath through your nose, and consciously follow it all the way through your respiratory system. Imagine the breath traveling deep into your abdomen. Then slowly release the breath and visualize it leaving your body. Repeat this process at least five times.

**2. Progressive relaxation** – this technique consciously tenses the muscles in the body, working from the feet to the head, in an effort to release the tension, leaving you relaxed. Starting with your feet, clench your muscles for five seconds and then release them. Move up to your calves and repeat. Work your way up to the crown of your head clenching and relaxing the major muscles in your body. By the end, you will notice all of your muscles will be more relaxed then when you started.

**3. Nasal awareness breathing** – Take deep breaths and focus on the sensation the air causes as it moves through your nose, from the tip all the way back to the throat. Repeat for several breathing cycles. An added benefit of Nasal Awareness Breathing prior to eating is that the scents of the food you are about to eat will help get the digestive juices flowing.

**4. Thanksgiving meditation** – If you are seated and ready to eat your meal, you have much to be grateful for. Take a moment to quiet your mind, breathe deeply, and give thanks for the abundance in your life. Let your thanksgiving practice spread to other areas of your life as well.

Once you are relaxed, focus on being thankful for the food you are about to eat. Be grateful that you *have* food and you are able to enjoy it. Let's face it, not everyone experiences that privilege. This will put your nervous system in the best possible state for digestion, and accepting the nutrients you are about to receive. While eating, try to extend the above awareness exercises into your eating process. Try to engage in "mindful eating" and bring your full awareness to the eating process: the act of chewing, the act of tasting, the act of smelling, etc. Really engage your senses. The more you engage your senses, the more parasympathetic activity will be engaged, and the better your digestion will be.

Another simple, but powerful, thing to remember is that the temperature of your water or beverages you consume will affect the mucus membranes and muscles they touch. Think of what a heating pad versus an ice pack does to your back muscles, the heat relaxes the muscles while the ice contracts them. The same is true with the fluids that come in contact with your digestive muscles. Having supple relaxed muscles goes hand and hand with peristaltic activity. Our internal body temperature is about 98 degrees so between 90°-98° is an ideal temperature for your beverages and foods -just be sure they are not too hot for your mouth.

## ENHANCING PARASYMPATHETIC ACTIVITY WITH BOTANICALS

There is a good chance that some people will need more help than a relaxation practice, or meditation, to facilitate their parasympathetic nervous system.

Using mediation in combination with the botanicals below can go a long way in relieving digestive issues related to inhibited peristaltic activity. The categories of herbs used to enhance parasympathetic activity are called *nervines*, *carminatives*, and *antispasmodics*. Consuming these herbs before, during, and after meals can help enhance parasympathetic activity. Let's look at some of the properties of these herbs.

A nervine has the property of calming nerves and activating parasympathetic activity. These can also be relaxing and help with sleeping too. Carminatives, on the other hand, enhance digestion by soothing the digestive tract, enhancing, digestive activity, and reducing and dispersing gas formation. Antispasmodics work like muscle relaxers to reduce spasms in the digestive muscles. The herbs mentioned below have a particular affinity for smooth muscle, which is the type of muscle in the digestive tract. As you will see below, many herbs will have a primary activity in one category and a secondary activity in other categories.

---

**TIP:  Eat quiet, , relaxed, meals while sitting down**
*Do not eat while driving, talking on the phone, or at your desk while you're working. Avoid noisy restaurants and upsetting conversations during meals if at all possible.*

---

## NERVINES

• **Chamomile** (*Matricaria chamomilla*) - Its primary activity is as a nervine and carminative, but it has mild antispasmodic properties as well. You can get chamomile tea from most major grocery stores. You can also buy the herb in bulk and make your own tea.

• **Scullcap** (*Scutellaria laterifolia*) – Primarily, skullcap is an antispasmodic but it also has strong nervine and sedative effects. This herb can be consumed in tincture form (alcohol extract) or tea. Finding this herb in bulk could be challenging.

• **Lemon Balm** (*Melissa officinalis*) – It is primarily a nervine with sedative and mild carminative effects. This can be found in some grocery stores as a pre-made tea bag. You may also be able to find it at specialty health food stores in bulk. Tea form is recommended unless it is in combination with other herbs.

## CARMINATIVES

• **Fennel** (*Foeniculum vulgare*) – Fennel is primarily a carminative with mild antispasmodic effects. You can actually find this in most grocery stores as it is a spice. You can make a tea out of the seeds or simply chew on the seeds before or after meals.

• **Anise** (*Pimpinella anisum*) - Anise is primarily a carminative and, like fennel, you can find this one at most grocery stores. The seed is the part that has the carminative effects and you can chew on them before or after meals to assist with digestion. This is often offered in Indian restaurants for a before and after meal digestive aid.

## ANTI-SPASMODICS

• **Crampbark** (*Viburnum opulus*)- It is primarily an antispasmodic but it also has nervine effects. It also has affinity to the uterus.

• **Wild Yam** ( *Diascorea villosa* ) – Primarily, wild yam is an antispasmodic but it also has a nervine effects with affinity to the digestive tract.

• **Hops** (*Humulus lupulus*)- Primarily, hops are used for their antispasmodic activity with an affinity for the digestive tract. They also has a sedative effect and contains nervine properties.

## EFFECTIVE CONSUMPTION OF HERBS

There are often specific relationships between what we eat and how it is absorbed in the body. These relationships can be good or bad. For example, dairy products can block the absorption of Iron, while Vitamin C boosts iron absorption. In the above example, Vitamin C and Iron have a synergistic relationship. The same kinds of relationships can exist between herbs and their effects on our bodies.

Using single herbs can be helpful but often, for the best results they should be combined with other herbs that support the desired effects of the primary herb. The process of herb combination is an art and is referred to as *herbal formulation*. Most herbs should be consumed in combination with other herbs that work synergistically with the primary herbs and the desired function. Typically herbal formulas are created specifically for an individual.

**An example case and herbal formula:**
*A woman with cramping pain, loose stools, and diarrhea that is worse with menstrual cycles and stress. She has difficulty sleeping and poor appetite during her menses as well.*
*25% Crampbark*
*30% Wild yam*
*15% Chamomile*
*15% Scullcap*
*10% Schizandra (overall balancing herb)*
*5% Cinnamon (for increased blood movement)*

**OTHER TREATMENTS**
Another technique to improve the peristaltic activity in your digestion is to use a rolled up warm towel or a warm water bottle directly on the abdomen. Roll it in a circular and clockwise motion lightly and gently. The heat will help the muscles relax, rather than spasm, and the pressure and motion will assist in the mechanical digestion of your food. This technique is especially helpful for those who are constipated as it helps to move the food through the digestive tract.

Along the lines of constipation, sitting in a squatting position first thing in the morning after eating - this is when the energy in the colon is most active - stretches the colon and improves the position for moment of food through the digestive tract. This stretching activity will actually have a slight pulling effect on the contents of the colon, assisting in a bowel movement. Sitting like this for three to five minutes during or after a meal, along with drinking lots of water and eating a diet high in fiber, is suggested for those who suffer from regular constipation. Often, your colon needs to be retrained. Once it becomes regular again, less effort is needed.

## 4. COLONIC BACTERIA
**What's the big deal with those "friendly bacteria" anyway?**

We have talked a little bit already about *probiotics*, or the friendly bacteria, that assist with the digestive process, **how they actually work will be the subject of this section.**

Information regarding *how* these small bacteria have such a big impact on digestion is only now beginning to be uncovered as more research emerges. One such discovery involves what occurs when certain bacterial strains overpopulate the large intestine (colon). This overpopulation by one strain is referred to as *dysbiosis* and leads to putrefaction, fermentation, and the release of gases that alter digestive function (discussed in detail below). The positive attributes of these bacteria come about from rebalancing any dysbiosis present. In this section we will explore the negative consequences of dysbiosis, and how certain probiotic strains can improve digestion by positively altering dysbiosis.

## THE NORMAL ECOLOGY OF THE LARGE INTESTINE

The large intestine is comprised of thousands of different strains of bacteria and other microorganisms (yeast, viruses, etc). There are actually more bacteria in your large intestine than there are cells in your body. In a healthy person, 80% or more of these bacteria are friendly and about 20% are unfriendly or *pathogenic*. I like to think about the large intestine as an isolated ecosystem, like a rain forest or high alpine environment. Using this analogy, the different strains of microorganisms make up the ecology of the system. When this local ecology is in harmony, there is a healthy, and sometimes symbiotic, relationship between the microorganisms, the cells of the digestive tract, called *enterocytes*, and the immune cells.

For example, the presence of the friendly bacteria suppresses the proliferation of the unfriendly or pathogenic bacteria by competing for space and food. The local immune system around the digestive tract, referred to as GALT (Gut Associated Lymphatic Tissue), also keeps the pathogenic microorganisms in check. In this way, both the friendly bacteria and the immune system keep the small amounts of pathogenic bacteria in check.

## HOW DOES THE BODY KNOW WHICH BACTERIA ARE FRIENDLY AND WHICH ARE NOT?

The immune system that surrounds the digestive tract has a unique relationship with the friendly bacteria that inhabit the colon. It is unclear exactly how this relationship develops but it appears as if the bacteria communicate with the immune cells. It is thought that the initial relationship starts shortly after birth, as the baby passes through the vaginal canal, as well as from ingestion of the mother's colostrum and breast milk.

When babies are born, there are no bacteria in their colons. However, as they pass through the vaginal canal, the baby ingests the bacteria that are present. The baby's colon is then inoculated with these bacteria.  As the baby's immune system develops, the bacteria in the colon develops along with it. The immune system only becomes alarmed when new bacteria, virus, fungus, or parasites are introduced. A quick side note: part of the natural inoculation process includes the colonization of fungi, like candida, as well.

These microorganisms feed on the passing unabsorbed fibrous food in proportion to their numbers. As they feed on this unabsorbed food, the bacteria excrete waste, which is called *butyrate*. This feeds and nourishes the enterocytes of the digestive tract, and also stimulates the enterocytes to grow and reproduce. There is also evidence suggesting these healthy bacteria assist with the enzymatic activity occurring inside the microvilli of the enterocytes. While these symbiotic relationships create a harmonious living environment among the bacteria and enterocytes, some bacteria can overgrow, creating disharmony. This disharmony is the dysbiosis referred to above.

Dysbiosis is the dysfunctional living environment created between two or more organisms. This can occur when one species, whether pathogenic *or* friendly, overpopulates and crowds out its neighbors. As this occurs the species will take more of the available resources and proliferate further. This snowball effect disrupts the inherent checks and balances in the colonic ecosystem.

**So what starts the disruption to begin with?** Do antibiotics affect the ecosystem? Do certain foods affect it?

We will look at these, and other questions, in more detail below.

## THE CAUSES OF DYSBIOSIS
### The effect of antibiotics

You might be surprised to learn that most antibiotics don't actually kill bacteria. It's true. Most antibiotics work by preventing the replication of bacteria, rather than killing them. Some antibiotics are specific for certain strains of bacteria and others are general, decreasing the replication of many different strains. In this way, when you take an antibiotic for a sickness in your lungs, most of the time you are effecting the bacteria in your large intestine too. The antibiotic stops the replication of the sensitive bacterial strains in the large intestine, allowing others that are not sensitive to overpopulate and overcrowd the colon. If the overgrowing bacteria are pathogenic strains, it can lead to severe problems - like in the case of *pseudomembranous colitis*.

Pseudomembranous colitis is caused by a relative excess of the bacteria *Cclostridium difficle*. The result of this severe intestinal infection is an uncontrollably severe diarrhea. In elderly and debilitated people, this infection can even lead to death from loss of fluid and sepsis. Sepsis occurs when bacteria enter into the blood stream and rapidly spread throughout the body. In the intestine, this happens from severe inflammation that leads to opening of the gap junctions between the intestinal cells. These openings allow the food and bacteria to seep into the blood stream. Of course, dysbiosis does not always cause such a severe outcome. Depending on how bad the dysbioisis is you may simply have a lot of extra gas.

## THE EFFECT OF TRANSIT TIME / EXCESS CARBS AND PROTEIN

In other cases of dysbiosis, the overgrowing bacteria create gases that lead to altered digestive flow. This alteration can either decrease or increase the flow of food through the digestive tract. The altered flow is not isolated to the large intestine. Because the gases can move through the digestive tract, it can alter digestion in the stomach and small intestine as well. Increased flow through the small intestine causes poor absorption, as there is insufficient time to breakdown and absorb the food. With poor carbohydrate breakdown and absorption in the small intestine, the large portions of carbohydrates enter the large intestine and amplify the issue further. The excess carbohydrates feed the already overpopulated bacterial species.

On the other hand decreased flow through the large intestine can also amplify the issue of dysbiosis as it gives the now overpopulating strains more feeding time. The bacteria typically have a limited amount of time to assist with the digestion of complex carbohydrates, leaving the remainder for waste. So *increased* time to feed can create problems too.

The transit time of foods through the digestive tract can be altered by drugs and medications too. Coffee, for instance, decreases transit time while codeine and other opiates increase transit time. Small infrequent changes in transit times will not usually alter the ecology of the colon. However chronic and ongoing changes will lead to problems.

**Now that we have covered the common *causes* of dysbiosis, let's explore the problems *created* by dysbiosis.**

_____

## TIP:  Drink enough water

*Adults should drink at least three quarts of water daily. Not drinking enough water can lead to constipation, which can lead to an out-pouching in the intestine. This can become inflamed and irritated leading to diverticulits.*

_____

## HEALTH ISSUES AND DYSBIOSIS

Dysbiosis leads to fermentation, production of disrupting gases, and putrefaction, all of which can have negative health consequences. The fermentation of carbohydrates by the overgrown bacteria creates alcohols and gases. These alcohols and gases are then absorbed into the blood stream and cause problems, both locally and systemically. Like any alcohol, the alcohol created by the bacteria are toxic to your body. The gases often cause discomfort and pain in the abdomen because they lead to changes in peristaltic activity (increases or decreases). This change can be the cause of chronic diarrhea or constipation (more on this below).

With fermentation and rampant overgrowth, the bacteria that are supposed to be isolated to the large intestine flow up into the small intestine. In normal conditions, there is little to no bacteria present in the small intestine. In cases where bacteria enter into the small intestine, they compete with your body for the carbohydrates and produce large amounts of gas. This fermentation in the small intestine creates one of two gases: hydrogen or methane. These gases interact with the muscles of the digestive tract changing the movement of foods. Hydrogen gas tends to produce diarrhea or loose stools, while methane produces constipation. Both gases can also produce bloating and pain. These gases can be tested for with a specific breath test. When an individual tests positive for one of these gases, they are thought to have a condition known as small intestinal bacterial overgrowth (SIBO). SIBO is emerging as a probable cause of many digestive disorders which previously went undiagnosed and / or had poor treatment options, such as IBS.  Testing and treatment for SIBO are relatively inexpensive considering cost of medication(that generally don't work well when you have SIBO) and the pain and suffering that comes along with this condition.

## PUTREFACTION

When proteins enter the large intestine it leads to a process called putrefaction. Putrefaction occurs in any setting where bacteria break down proteins. The process involved in the decomposition of an animal is an example of putrefaction. The terrible smell  associated with that process is produced by the chemicals created when bacteria break down proteins. When it happens in the large intestine of our body, it can lead to very harmful and toxic substances that are absorbed into the body. As the bacteria break down the proteins, they release harmful byproducts like *putrescine* and *cadaverine*. These are both *neurotoxic*, toxic to the nerves, and *cytotoxic*, toxic to the cells, causing health issues like inflammation, headaches, pain, confusion, foggy thinking, and more - both locally and systemically.

## HOW DO I KNOW IF I HAVE DYSBIOSIS OR OTHER PROBLEMS WITH INTESTINAL BACTERIA?

More than likely you do have a little dysbiosis. How much of a "problem" it is will vary based on the influences mentioned above. More serious cases include the following symptoms:
• Gas and bloating two hours after meals (can also be insufficient pancreatic enzymes),
• Feeling sick after meals,
• Getting headaches close to or after meals
• Unexplainable fatigue, headaches
• Diagnosis of IBS, Crohn's, Ulcerative Colitis
• Unexplained constipation, diarrhea, or abdominal pain.

_____

### TIP: Toxins in food

*Dough conditioners, MSG, sweeteners like aspartame and sugar, artificial colors, artificial flavors, pesticides and insecticides are all toxins. The US government allows more than 3000 of these toxins to be added to our foods. Read labels, especially when consuming packaged foods.*

_____

Of course, the best way to know for sure if you have dysbiosis is to have some testing done. There are tests that measure the types, and quantity, of bacteria present in the colon. You can also test for hydrogen or methane gases. For most of these tests you will need both an initial *and* follow up visit to a knowledgeable doctor. It is likely that you can make a good judgment call based on the influences and symptoms mentioned above. However, having someone guide you along the way can make a big difference because the symptoms can all seem the same, making differentiation difficult. The good news is that the treatments below will not be harmful to your system. Doing a few therapeutic trials can go a long way to giving you some clues as to what is wrong and put you on the track to better health.

### WHAT CAN I DO TO TREAT MY DYSBIOSIS PROBLEMS?

First things first: treat the cause. Probiotics are probably the quickest and easiest way to improve the biotic environment of your large intestine. While the market is flooded with different probiotics, there are two species that seem to have the most consistently positive correlations to improved digestive function. It's worth noting that I have found these two strains to work favorably in my patients as well.

These strains are:
• *Lactobacillus acidophilus*
• *Bifidobacteria bifidus*

You should know that these are not the only strains that are known to be helpful. Numerous studies have shown other species to have favorable improvements in digestive function. The ones mentioned above have consistent positive result in research and clinical use. I suggest you start with the *Lactobacillus acidophilus* and *Bifidobacterium bifidus*. The dose you should take is between 2-5 billion total bacteria one to two times daily.  Sometimes more than this can be helpful for short periods of time.  An effective treatment trial for dysbiosis would be about three to six weeks. If there is improvement in this time frame, you can expect any further improvements to be very small. This is, of course, if your diet is free of foods, drinks and medicines that would perpetuate the dysbiosis during this time.

## *A NOTE ON PROBIOTICS*

*Some probiotic supplements also add what is known as a **prebiotic**. Prebiotics are the disaccharides (small carbohydrate) that the colonic bacteria preferentially eat. Prebiotics are usually not necessary but can be marginally helpful. In addition to oral probiotics, other fermented foods like yogurt, sauerkraut, and kimchee, can be helpful as well.*

*If these don't help, consider adding Saccharomyces boulardi, which is a yeast that can help balance the bacteria and yeast in the colon and improve the symptoms mentioned above. 1-2 billion daily should be sufficient.*

## DIET FOR DYSBIOSIS

The diet to improve dysbiosis is a diet low in refined carbohydrates. Even small amounts of sugary foods entering the large intestine will sabotage any effort to rebalance this delicate ecology.  A Paleolithic-type diet would be advised during the three to six week period. A paleolithic diet is one that has very little grains. It consists of nuts, berries, fruits, veggies, and lean meats. This diet is also free of any dairy products. This is the type of diet our ancestors lived on before we started cultivating grains. The friendly bacteria in our digestive tract likely evolved with us and are more adapted to this "paleo" diet.

You should also be eating plenty of fibrous foods as these feed the good bacteria. Fermented foods like yogurt, kimchee, and sauerkraut, can also be helpful. These foods have good bacteria in them as well. They are not as potent as the probiotics but are still very helpful.

## SUMMARY

There were many digestive topics covered here, from the basics of how things work, to what to do when something is amiss with your digestive system. To summarize, let me just say:

• Without digestive enzymes the foods we eat will not be broken down into their smaller counterparts, and absorption of the corresponding nutrients is limited. Decreased acid production in the stomach leads to decreased activation of enzymes. There are several steps that can be taken to increase acid production and enzyme activation for complete food break down.

• Your intestinal mucosa is a delicate make up of fine absorptive projections that capture nutrients from the lumen. When these projections are limited from damage or otherwise, the absorptive capacity of the small intestine is impaired. Repairing the damage, reducing inflammation, and removing the causes of inflammation, are important players in maintaining and restoring mucosal health.

• The intestinal nervous system is reactive to the "actual" external environment and the "perceived" external environment. Even if you are in a calm physical place, if you feel stress, these feelings are transmitted through the nervous system and into the digestive tract. The effects of stress on digestion are counteractive to the break down and absorption of nutrients. In order to get the most out of the foods you eat, you have to nourish the parasympathetic activity that is integral to the digestive process. Relaxation techniques can be helpful to this nourishing process.

• The many species of bacteria that populate our colon play an integral part of food breakdown, immune system activation, and more. These bacteria live in a delicate balance and any disruption in that balance creates problems locally and systemically. Achieving and maintaining this balance is needed for optimal digestion.

As you can see digestion is more than a simple mechanical process. It requires a coordination of efforts from different systems in the body. When the coordination is in sync, digestion of food delivers nourishment of vitamins, minerals, and other nutrients to the cells of the body. This nourishment provides energy to the body's cells, helps soothe inflammation, and improves efficiency of all cellular processes. Without good digestion, the rest of the body will not be able to perform at its best. If you have digestive system problems, follow the instructions in this book and your digestion will improve.

## ABOUT DR. ROBIN TERRANELLA

Doctor Terranella has been practicing integrative medicine for 6 years in Phoenix Arizona. Over this time he has treated a wide variety of health issues, many of which are direct related to digestive function. Digestion is interrelated to so many aspects of health, he believes it to be one of the core foundations of health. We have all heard how exercise and good diet are essential to health. Because our digestion feeds the rest of our bodies with nutrients it is just as important as diet and exercise. Countless books have been written on diet and exercise but proportionally very few on digestion.

As he has observed in many of his patients, many people don't know how important digestion is and how it is connected to other areas of health. So much can be done by healing and improving the health of our digestion. That's why he felt compelled to share this information with the world.

Doctor Terranella attended medical school at Bastyr University and received a doctorate of Naturopathic Medicine in 2006. He also received a degree in Acupuncture from Wu Hsing Tao. He has been practicing integrative medicine since 2007.

www.ingramcontent.com/pod-product-compliance
Lightning Source LLC
Chambersburg PA
CBHW060213290526
45789CB00003B/1246

*9 7 8 1 5 0 0 3 0 4 4 0 9 *